Mediterranean Diet for Beginners:

100 Weight Loss Recipes for Healthy Living and a 4-Week Meal Plan

Table of contents

Week 1

Include a snack of your choice during the day when you get hungry. If you don't feel hungry between meals, skip it.

Day 1

Breakfast Couscous

Ingredients

Butter (4 tsp. melted, divided)

Salt (.25 tsp.)

Raw sugar (6 tsp. divided)

Currants (.25 cups dried)

Apricots (.5 cups)

Couscous (1 cup)

Cinnamon stick (2-inch)

Low-fat milk (3 cups)

How's it Made

In a large saucepan, add in the cinnamon stick as well as the milk before placing the saucepan on a burner turned to a high/medium heat. Let it cook for 3 minutes but do not let it boil.

Remove the saucepan from the stove before adding in the salt, 4 tsp. brown sugar, the currants, apricots and couscous.

Cover the pan and let it rest for 15 minutes.

Remove the cinnamon stick, add in the remaining butter and sugar to taste, serve warm and enjoy.

Greek Salad

Ingredients

Red onion (.5 sliced)

Sun dried tomatoes (.3 cups)

Roma tomatoes (3 cups diced)

Black olives (1 cup sliced)

Feta cheese (1.5 cups)

Cucumber (3 sliced)

How's it Made

Combine all of the ingredients, and mix well to coat.

Chill, serve and enjoy.

Meat Pies

Ingredients

Puff pastry sheet (1 halved)

Egg (1 beaten)

Lemon juice (.3 cups)

Salt and pepper (to taste)

Cinnamon (to taste)

Pine nuts (.75 cups)

White onion (1 chopped)

Lamb (.5 lbs. ground)

Beef (.5 lbs. ground)

How's it Made

Coat a pan in the oil and place it on the stove above a burner that has been turned to a high/medium heat.

Add in the meat as well as the salt and pepper, cinnamon, pine nuts and onion.

Let the meat cook completely before adding in the lemon juice and letting the meat cool.

Ensure your oven is heated to 350 degrees.

Line a baking sheet with parchment paper.

Prepare the puff pastry before adding the meat to the middle.

Add pies to baking sheet before brushing each with egg wash.

Cook for 15 minutes, serve hot and enjoy.

Day 2

Potato Hash with Chickpeas

Ingredients

Eggs (4)

Zucchini (1 cup chopped)

Chickpeas (15 oz. can)

Olive oil (.25 cups)

Salt (.5 tsp.)

Curry powder (1 T)

Ginger (1 T minced)

Onion (.5 cups chopped)

Baby spinach (2 cups chopped)

Potatoes (4 cups shredded)

How's it Made

In a large bowl, add the salt, curry powder, ginger, onion, spinach and potatoes.

Coat a pan in the oil and place it on the stove above a burner that has been turned to a high/medium heat.

Add in the mixture from the bowl and pack it down firmly before letting it cook for 3 minutes.

Turn the heat to low/medium before adding in the zucchini and chickpeas and breaking up the potato mixture until everything is mixed well.

Press down on the results firmly, leaving 4 holes for the eggs to occupy.

Add in eggs and let everything cook 4 additional minutes.

Serve hot and enjoy.

Baked Falafel

Ingredients

Olive oil (2 tsp.)

Egg (1 beaten)

Flour (1 T)

Baking soda (.25 tsp.)

Salt (.25 tsp.)

Coriander (.25 tsp.)

Cumin (1 tsp.)

Garlic (3 cloves minced)

Parsley (.25 cups chopped)

Garbanzo beans (15 oz. drained)

Onion (.25 cups chopped)

How's it Made

In a food processor, add in the baking soda, salt, coriander, cumin, garlic, parsley and garbanzo beans and process well.

Add the results to a bowl before mixing in the onion, egg and flour.

Shape the results into patties and let them set for 15 minutes.

Ensure your oven is preheated to 400 degrees Fahrenheit.

Coat a pan in the oil and place it on the stove above a burner that has been turned to a high/medium heat.

Add the patties to the skillet and let each side cook for 3 minutes.

Add the skillet to the oven and let the patties cook an additional 10 minutes.

Serve hot and enjoy.

Balsamic Chicken

Ingredients

Thyme (.5 tsp. dried)

Rosemary (1 tsp. dried)

Basil (1 tsp. dried)

Balsamic vinegar (.5 cups)

Tomatoes (14.5 oz. can diced)

Onion (1 sliced)

Olive oil (2 T)

Pepper (to taste)

Garlic salt (1 tsp.)

Chicken breast (3 halved)

How's it made

Add seasoning to chicken as desired.

Coat a pan in the oil and place it on the stove above a burner that has been turned to a medium heat.

Let each side of the chicken cook for 3 minutes before mixing in the onion and letting it cook for 3 minutes.

Add in the vinegar and tomatoes before adding the thyme, rosemary, oregano and basil. Cover the pan and let the chicken simmer for 15 minutes.

The chicken's internal temperature should read 165 degrees Fahrenheit.

Serve hot and enjoy.

Day 3

Avocado Toast

Ingredients

Rye bread (4 slices)

Lemon juice (to taste)

Mint (2 T chopped)

Feta cheese (80 grams crumbled)

Avocados (2, peeled, pitted)

Pepper (to taste)

Salt (to taste)

How's it Made

Mash the avocado using a fork in a medium-sized bowl.

Mix in the lemon juice and mint and mix well before adding the pepper and salt as needed.

Toast the bread, add the avocado and top with the mint, serve warm and enjoy.

Quinoa Salad

Ingredients

Olive oil (.25 cups)

Balsamic vinegar (1 T)

Lemon juice (.6 cups)

Salt (.5 tsp.)

Chives (.25 cups)

Parsley (.25 cups)

Feta cheese (.5 cups)

Kalamata olives (.5 cups chopped)

Green bell pepper (1 diced)

Chicken breast (2 cooked, cubed)

Quinoa (1 cup)

Garlic (1 clove smashed)

Chicken bouillon (2 cubes)

Water (2 cups)

How's it Made

Add the garlic, bouillon and water to a saucepan and bring the pan to a boil.

Add in the quinoa and turn the burner to low/medium to let it simmer for 15 minutes with the pan covered.

Remove the garlic and add the quinoa from the bot to a large bowl.

Add in the salt, chives, parsley, feta cheese, olive, bell pepper, onion and chicken before topping with the olive oil, vinegar and lemon juice.

Serve and enjoy.

Greek Sea Bass

Ingredients

Lemon wedges (2)

Italian flat-leaf parsley (.25 cups)

Oregano leaves (1 T)

Lemon juice (.25 cups)

White wine (.5 cups)

Rosemary (2 sprigs)

Sea bass (2 cleaned)

Pepper and salt (to taste)

Red onion (1 chopped)

Olive oil (2 T divided)

How's it made

Ensure your oven is preheated to 325 degrees Fahrenheit.

Coat a baking pan in half of the olive oil before adding the pepper, salt and onion.

Add the fish to the pan after placing red onion, rosemary and lemon in each. Top with oregano, lemon juice and white wine before adding the remaining olive oil.

Add the baking pan to the oven and let the fish cook for 25 minutes.

Serve hot and enjoy.

Day 4

Greek Pancakes

Ingredients

Canola oil (2 T)

Agave (2 T)

Eggs (2)

Greek Yogurt (2 cups)

Salt (.25 tsp.)

Baking soda (1 tsp.)

Flax seeds (2 T)

Flour (.5 cups)

Rolled oats (1 cup)

How's it Made

Mix the rolled oats, flour, flax seeds, baking soda and salt together in a blender and process for half a minute.

Mix in the agave, oil, eggs and yogurt and combine well. Let the results sit for 20 minutes.

Coat a pan in the oil and place it on the stove above a burner that has been turned to a high/medium heat.

Add batter to the pan at the rate of .25 cups per pancake.

Let each side of each pancake cook for 2 minutes before adding them to a cooking sheet to keep them warm during the cooking process.

Serve warm and enjoy.

Mediterranean Kale

Ingredients

Salt and pepper (to taste)

Soy sauce (1 tsp.)

Garlic (1 T minced)

Olive oil (1 T)

Lemon juice (2 T)

Kale (12 cups chopped)

How's it Made

Steam the kale

Combine the salt and pepper together along with the soy sauce, garlic olive oil and lemon juice.

Add the kale to the bowl and mix well to coat.

Serve warm and enjoy.

Mediterranean Chicken

Ingredients

.25 cups water

Cornstarch (1.5 tsp.)

Salt (.5 tsp.)

Sour cream (.5 cups)

Parsley (2 T)

Dry white wine (.5 cups)

Green olives (2 T sliced)

Sun dried tomatoes (.25 cups chopped)

Italian seasoning (1 T)

Black pepper (.5 tsp.)

Salt (.5 tsp.)

Garlic (3 cloves minced)

Chicken tenders (12)

Olive oil (2 T)

How's it Made

Coat a pan in the oil and place it on the stove above a burner that has been turned to a high/medium heat.

Add the garlic and chicken to the pan followed by the seasoning, pepper, salt, tomatoes, parsley, win and olives.

Turn the heat to a low setting and let the chicken cook completely. The chicken's internal temperature should read 165 degrees Fahrenheit.

Remove the chicken before adding the milk and sour cream to the pan.

In a small bowl, combine the water and cornstarch.

Raise the heat on the pan to medium before adding in the water and cornstarch.

Stir the sauce until it is the desired thickness, add sauce to chicken, serve hot and enjoy.

Day 5

Frittata

Ingredients

Basil leaves (crushed, to taste)

Parmesan cheese (2 T)

Croutons (.5 cups crushed)

Pepper (to taste)

Salt (to taste)

Green olives (.5 cups sliced, pitted)

Roasted red sweet peppers (.5 cup bottled)

Feta cheese (2 oz.)

Light cream (.25 cups)

Eggs (8 beaten)

Olive oil (3 T)

Garlic (2 cloves minced)

Onion (1 cup chopped)

How's it Made

Ensure your broiler is fully heated.

Coat a pan in 2 T of the oil and place it on the stove above a burner that has been turned to a high/medium heat.

Add in the garlic as well as the onion and let them cook until the onion is tender.

Combine the pepper, salt, basil, olives, roasted red peppers, feta cheese, light cream, and eggs in a large bowl.

Add the results to the skillet after turning it to a medium heat.

Let the eggs cook, making sure to rotate eggs regularly to ensure an even texture.

Mix the remainder of the oil, parmesan cheese and croutons together in a small bowl before adding the results to the egg mixture.

Place the pan beneath the broiler at about 6 inches and let it cook for an additional 1 minute.

Serve hot and enjoy.

Hummus and Pita

Ingredients

Olive oil (2 T)

Sal/pepper (to taste)

Garlic (1 clove chopped)

Tahini (2 T)

Lemon juice (4 T)

Garbanzo beans (19 oz. half liquid retained)

Garlic (1 clove)

Pita to (taste)

How's it Made

Place all ingredients into a blender and blend until smooth.

Serve with pita and enjoy.

Flounder with Kalamata Olives

Ingredients

Basil leaves (6 torn)

Flounder fillets (1 lb.)

Parmesan cheese (3 T grated)

Lemon juice (1 tsp.)

Capers (.25 cups)

White wine (.25 cups)

Kalamata olives (pitted, chopped)

Italian seasoning (1 pinch)

Garlic (2 cloves chopped)

Spanish onion (.5 chopped)

Olive oil (2 T)

Roma tomatoes (5)

How's it Made

Ensure the oven has been preheated to 425 degrees Fahrenheit.

Add water to a saucepan and place it on a burner turned to a high heat and let it boil.

Add in the tomatoes for 10 seconds before removing them and placing them in cold water to stop them from cooking. Chop and peel the tomatoes.

Coat a pan in the oil and place it on the stove above a burner that has been turned to a medium heat.

Add the onions and let them cook for 5 minutes.

Add in the seasoning, garlic and tomatoes and let everything cook for 5 minutes.

Add in the basil, lemon juice, capers, wine and olives before turning the heat to low.

Add in the parmesan cheese and let everything cook for 15 minutes.

Add the fish to a baking dish before topping with sauce.

Let the fish bake for 12 minutes, serve hot and enjoy.

Day 6

Banana Oatmeal

Ingredients

Banana (1 peeled)

Honey (3 T)

Walnuts (2 T chopped)

Flax seeds (1 tsp.)

Skim milk (.5 cups)

Rolled oats (.25 cups)

How's it Made

In a microwaveable bowel, mix the banana, honey, walnuts, flax seeds, milk and oats together before microwaving them on a normal setting for 2 minutes.

Mash the banana and stir well, serve hot and enjoy.

Greek Chicken Pasta

Ingredients

Pepper and salt (to taste)

Oregano (2 tsp.)

Lemon juice (2 T)

Parsley (3 T chopped)

Feta cheese (.5 cups crumbled)

Tomato (1 chopped)

Artichoke hearts (14 oz. chopped)

Chicken breasted (1 lb. cubed)

Garlic (2 cloves crushed)

Olive oil (1 T)

Red onion (.5 cups chopped)

Linguine pasta (16 oz.)

How's it Made

Add a pinch of salt and water to a large pot before letting the water come to a boil.

Mix in the pasta and let it cook for 8 minutes prior to draining.

Coat a pan in the oil and place it on the stove above a burner that has been turned to a high/medium heat.

Add in the garlic and onion and let them cook for 2 minutes.

Add in the chicken and let it cook for 5 minutes.

Turn the heat to low/medium before adding in the pasta, oregano, lemon juice, parsley, feta cheese, tomato and artichoke hearts and letting everything cook for 2 minutes.

Serve warm and enjoy.

Grecian Tilapia

Ingredients

Kalamata olives (2 T chopped, pitted)

Lemon juice (1 T)

Sun dried tomato oil (1 T)

Tilapia Fillets (2)

Capers (1 T)

Sun dried tomatoes (3 T)

How's it Made

Ensure your oven is preheated to 375 degrees Fahrenheit.

Combine the capers, olives and tomatoes together in a small bowl.

In a baking dish, add the tilapia before topping with lemon juice and tomato oil.

Add the fish to the oven and let it bake for 10 minutes.

Add tomatoes to the fish, serve and enjoy.

Day 7

Veggie Omelet

Ingredients

Parsley (2 T chopped)

Goat cheese (.5 cups crumbled)

Pepper (.5 tsp.)

Salt (.25 tsp.)

Eggs (6)

Artichoke hearts (.25 cups, chopped)

Green olives (.25 cups pitted, chopped)

Roma tomato (1 diced)

Olive oil (1 T)

How's it Made

Ensure your oven is heated to 325 degrees Fahrenheit

Coat a pan in the oil and place it on the stove above a burner that has been turned to a high/medium heat.

Mix in the fennel and let it cook for 5 minutes.

Mix in the artichoke hearts, olives and tomato and cook for 3 minutes.

In a large bowl, whisk pepper, salt and eggs together.

Add the eggs to the pan and let it cook for 2 minutes.

Add cheese and let it cook for 5 minutes.

Add parsley, serve hot and enjoy.

Mediterranean Fish

Ingredients

Lemon juice (1 T)

Pepper (to taste)

Salt (to taste)

Olive oil (.25 cups)

Capers (.25 cups)

Kalamata olives (5 oz.)

Onion (1 chopped)

Tomato (1 chopped)

Greek seasoning (1 T)

Halibut filets (4, 6 oz.)

How's it Made

Ensure your oven is preheated to 350 degrees Fahrenheit.

Add the halibut to aluminum foil before adding the seasoning.

In a mixing bowl, add the pepper, salt, lemon juice, olive oil, capers, olives, onion, and tomato before adding it to the halibut.

Encase the results in foil and add to a baking sheet.

Let the fish bake for 30 minutes.

Serve hot and enjoy.

Sautéed Chicken

Ingredients

Pepper and salt (to taste)

Parsley (.25 cups chopped)

Kalamata olives (.5 cups, pitted, sliced)

Basil (1 T chopped)

Thyme (2 tsp. chopped)

White wine (.5 cups)

Tomatoes (3 cups chopped0

Onion (.5 cups diced)

Garlic (3 cloves minced)

Chicken breast (3 halved)

White wine (2 T)

Olive oil (2 tsp.)

How's it Made

Coat a pan in the oil and 2 T wine and place it on the stove above a burner that has been turned to a high/medium heat.

Add the chicken and let each side cook for 4 minutes.

Remove the chicken before adding the garlic and letting it cook for 30 seconds before mixing in the onion and letting them both cook for 3 minutes.

Mix in the tomatoes before letting the pan boil.

After it has boiled, turn the heat to low/medium and add in the remainder of the wine, let it cook for 10 minutes, mix in the basil and thyme and let everything cook for 5 more minutes.

Add the chicken back to the skillet, cover the pan and let the chicken cook until it reaches an internal temperature of 165 degrees Fahrenheit.

Mix in the parsley and olives before cooking for 1 final minute.

Season, serve hot and enjoy.

Week 2

I nclude a snack of your choice during the day when you get hungry. If you don't feel hungry between meals, skip it.

Day 1

Goat Cheese/Zucchini Frittata

Ingredients

Goat cheese (2 oz.)

Garlic (1 clove)

Olive oil (1 T)

Pepper (to taste)

Salt (.25 tsp.)

Milk (2 T)

Eggs (8)

Zucchinis (2 sliced)

How's it Made

Ensure your oven is preheated to 350 degrees.

Combine the pepper, salt, milk and eggs together in a large bowl.

Coat a pan in the oil and place it on the stove above a burner that has been turned to a high/medium heat.

Add in the zucchini and garlic and let them sauté for 5 minutes.

Add in the eggs and stir well for 60 seconds.

Remove the pan from the stove, top frittata with cheese and bake for 10 minutes.

Let it cool for 3 minutes, serve warm and enjoy.

Barley Salad

Ingredients

Olive oil (2 T)

Black olives (4 oz. chopped)

Cilantro (.5 cups chopped)

Balsamic vinegar (1 T)

Garlic (2 cloves)

Sun dried tomatoes (7)

Water (2.5 cups)

Barley (1 cup)

How's it Made

Add the water and barley to a saucepan before adding it to a burner turned to a high heat.

Once it boils, turn the heat to low/medium before letting it simmer, covered for 30 minutes. Let the barley drain then cool.

Add the vinegar, olive oil, garlic and tomatoes to a blender and blend well.

Add the results to the barley before adding the remaining ingredients and mixing well.

Refrigerate prior to serving.

Garlic-rubbed Salmon

Ingredients

Garlic salt (1.5 tsp.)

Basil (1 T chopped)

Cilantro (1 T chopped)

Salmon fillet (4, 3 oz. each)

Balsamic vinegar (.25 cups)

Olive oil (.5 cups)

How's it Made

In a small bowl, add the vinegar and olive oil and mix well.

Rub the fish with the garlic before adding to a baking dish and topping with the olive oil mixture.

Season as desired and let sit for 10 minutes.

Ensure your broiler is heated before placing the fish about 6 inches beneath it and letting it cook for 15 minutes, making sure to brush with sauce every 5 minutes to prevent dryness.

Serve hot and enjoy.

Day 2

Egg Scramble

Ingredients

Olive oil (5 tsp. divided)

Pepper/sat (to taste)

Eggs (6)

Ricotta cheese (.25 cups)

Parsley (.25 cups chopped)

Black olives (8 chopped)

Red pepper (.25 diced)

Potatoes (3 sliced)

Butter (1 tsp.)

How's it Made

Coat a pan in the oil, add in the butter and place it on the stove above a burner that has been turned to a high/medium heat.

Mix in the potatoes and let them cook for 15 minutes.

Mix in the olives and bell pepper and let everything cook for 4 minutes.

Combine the eggs, ricotta and parsley together in a mixing bowl.

Add the results to the pan and stirring regularly for 3 minutes.

Serve hot and enjoy.

Feta and Spinach Pita Bake

Ingredients

Pepper and salt (to taste)

Olive oil (3 T)

Parmesan cheese (2 T)

Feta cheese (.5 cups)

Mushrooms (4 sliced)

Spinach (1 bunch chopped)

Roma tomatoes (2 chopped)

Pita breads (6)

Tomato pesto (6 oz.)

How's it Made

Ensure your oven is preheated to 350 degrees Fahrenheit.

Add the pesto to the pita breads and lay them facing up on a baking sheet.

Add the olive oil, cheeses, mushrooms, spinach and tomatoes to the top of the pitta before seasoning as desired.

Add the baking sheet to the oven and bake for 12 minutes.

Serve hot and enjoy.

Chicken Sausage Skillet

Ingredients

Red grapes (.6 cups)

Almonds (.25 cups slivered)

Salt (.25 tsp.)

Basil (.3 cups chopped)

Plain Greek Yogurt (1 cup)

Parsley (1 T)

Sage (.25 tsp. ground)

Chicken broth (.5 cups)

Long grain rice (2 cups cooked)

Apricots (3 dried, chopped)

Scallions (.3 cups chopped)

Olive oil (1 T)

Chicken Sausage (12 oz. cooked, sliced)

How's it Made

Coat a pan in the oil and place it on the stove above a burner that has been turned to a high/medium heat.

Add in the scallions and let them cook for 3 minutes.

Mix in the apricots and sausage and the m them cook for 5 minutes.

Mix in the broth and the rice and let it simmer for 60 seconds before mixing in the parsley and sage and letting everything cook for an additional minute.

Mix in the grapes, remove from heat, season, top with almonds, serve and enjoy.

Day 3

Lemon Scones

Ingredients

Lemon juice (1 tsp.)

Powdered sugar (1 cup)

Buttermilk (.75 cups)

Lemon zest (1 lemon)

Butter (.25 cups)

Salt (.5 tsp.)

Baking soda (.5 tsp.)

Sugar (2 T)

Flour (2 cups +.25 cups)

How's it Made

Ensure the oven is heated to 400 degrees Fahrenheit.

Combine the salt, baking soda, sugar, and 2 cups flour together in a mixing bowl.

Add the results to a food processor, process, add in the butter and process until crumbles form.

Mix in the buttermilk and lemon zest.

Flour a surface and place the dough on top of it.

Prepare the dough to be baked, the dough should create 12 scones.

Add the scones to a baking sheet, add the baking sheet to the oven and cook for 12 minutes.

Mix lemon juice and powdered sugar together, add to scones, serve warm and enjoy.

Roasted Red Pepper Hummus

Ingredients

Parsley (1 T)

Salt (.25 tsp.)

Cayenne pepper (.5 tsp.)

Cumin (.5 tsp.)

Garlic (1 clove minced)

Tahini (1.5 T)

Lemon juice (3 T)

Roasted red peppers (4 oz.)

Garbanzo beans (15 oz. can)

Pita (to taste)

How's it Made

Add the salt, cayenne, cumin, garlic, tahini, lemon juice, red peppers and chickpeas together in a blender and blend well.

Keep in the refrigerator for 1 hour prior to serving, top with parsley, serve with pita and enjoy.

Sardine Casserole

Ingredients

Bread crumbs (2 T)

Basil (1 T)

Garlic (2 cloves chopped)

Cherry tomatoes (.5 lbs. diced)

Sardines (17.5 oz.)

Olive oil (3 T)

Russet potatoes (1 lb.)

How's it Made

Add the potatoes to a pot before covering them with salted water and letting the pot boil.

Once it boils, turn the heat to low/medium before placing a lid on it and letting the potatoes cook for 20 minutes.

Drain the potatoes and cover them in cold water to let them cool.

Slice and peel the potatoes.

Ensure your oven is heated to 350 degrees Fahrenheit.

Add the olive oil to a casserole dish and coat well.

Alternate layers of potato and layers of sardine, adding the tomatoes to the sardine layers. Top with bread crumbs, basil and garlic.

Let the casserole cook for 20 minutes, serve hot and enjoy.

Day 4

Pita Bread and Fava Beans

Ingredients

Pita bread pockets (4)

Lemon juice (.25 cups)

Parsley (.25 cups chopped)

Cumin (1 tsp. ground)

Fava beans (15 oz. can)

Garlic (1 clove crushed)

Tomato (1 diced)

Onion (1 chopped)

Olive oil (1.5 T)

How's it Made

Coat a pan in the oil and place it on the stove above a burner that has been turned to a high/medium heat.

Add in the garlic, tomato and onion and let them cook for 3 minutes.

Mix in the fava beans, including liquid and bring results to a boil.

Turn the heat to medium before adding in the lemon juice, parsley and cumin.

Let results continue cooking for 5 minutes

Heat pita, combine ingredients, serve warm and enjoy.

Grecian Potatoes

Ingredients

Potatoes (6 peeled, quartered)

Salt and pepper (to taste)

Chicken bouillon (2 cubes)

Rosemary (1 tsp.)

Thyme (1 tsp.)

Lemon juice (.25 cups)

Garlic (2 cloves)

Water (1.5 cups)

Olive oil (.3 cups)

How's it Made

Ensure your oven is preheated to 350 degrees Fahrenheit.

Combine the pepper, salt, bouillon cubes, rosemary, thyme, lemon juice, garlic, water and olive oil together in a small bowl.

Place the potatoes at the bottom of the baking dish before adding the olive oil.

Cover the dish and let it bake for 90 minutes, turning every 15 minutes.

Serve hot and enjoy.

Lamb Burger

Ingredients

Arugula (8 leaves)

Feta cheese (8 oz. sliced)

Ciabatta rolls (4 sliced)

Green tomato (1 sliced)

Sweet onion (1 sliced)

Salt (.5 tsp.)

Garlic (1 clove minced)

Lemon zest (1 lemon)

Plain Greek Yogurt (16 oz.)

Pepper (.5 tsp.)

Salt (1 tsp.)

Garlic (1 tsp. minced)

Ginger root (1 tsp. minced)

Mint (3 T chopped)

Lamb (1 lb. ground)

Beef (.5 lbs. ground)

How's it Made

Add oil to your grill and heat it to a high/medium heat.

In a large bowl, combine the pepper, tsp. salt, tsp. garlic, ginger, mint, beef and lamb together.

Portion out patties.

In a small bowl, combine the remaining salt, garlic, lemon zest and greet yogurt together and place in the refrigerator.

Place the patties on the grill and let them cook for 3 minutes on either side.

Add the buns to the grill and let each side cook for 60 seconds, grill vegetables as desired.

Combine ingredients, serve hot and enjoy.

Day 5

Breakfast Pita

Ingredients

Parsley (1 handful chopped)

Tomatoes (2 diced)

Cucumber (1 sliced)

Hummus (4 oz.)

Pita pockets (2)

Eggs (4)

How's it Made

Add water to a saucepan before letting it boil

Add in eggs and let them cook for 7 minutes

Peel the eggs and cut them into slices.

Add all ingredients together, serve warm and enjoy.

Garbanzo beans with Spinach

Ingredients

Salt (.5 tsp.)

Cumin (.5 tsp.)

Garbanzo beans (12 oz.)

Spinach (10 oz. chopped)

Onion (.5 diced)

Garlic (4 cloves minced)

Olive oil (1 T)

How's it Made

Coat a pan in the oil and place it on the stove above a burner that has been turned to a high/medium heat.

Add the onion and garlic to the pan and let it cook for 5 minutes.

Add in the salt, cumin, garbanzo beans and mash the beans partially before letting them cook fully.

Serve hot and enjoy.

Spaghetti Squash

Ingredients

Parsley (1 T chopped)

Tomato (1 chopped)

Lemon pepper (1 pinch)

Salt and pepper (to taste)

Feta cheese (4 oz.)

Italian seasoning (1 T)

Red bell pepper (1 diced)

Zucchini (1 diced)

Garlic (3 cloves minced)

Spring onions (2 chopped)

Italian sausage links (4 oz. casing removed)

Spaghetti squash (1 vertically halved, seeded)

Olive Oil (2 T)

How's it Made

Ensure your oven is heated to 350 degrees Fahrenheit.

Add half the olive oil to a baking dish and coat well.

Add the squash face down to the dish.

Add the dish to the oven and let it cook for 45 minutes before flipping the squash and letting the other side bake for 5 minutes.

Coat a pan in the oil and place it on the stove above a burner that has been turned to a medium heat.

Add the sausage and let it cook for 5 minutes before removing.

In the pan, mix in the seasoning, red peppers and zucchini before cooking 5 more minutes.

Add the cheese and the squash to the pan before cooking for 3 minutes

Combine all ingredients, serve warm and enjoy.

Day 6

Breakfast Sandwich

Ingredients

Tomato (1 slice)

Spinach leaves (.5 cups sliced)

Egg (1 cooked over easy)

Wheat toast (2 slices)

Butter (1 tsp.)

How's it made

Cook egg as desired.

Toast bread, combine ingredients, serve warm and enjoy.

Chicken Milano

Ingredients

Green beans (9 oz.)

Stewed tomatoes (28 oz. can)

Salt and pepper (to taste)

Red pepper flakes (1 tsp.)

Italian seasoning (1 tsp.)

Garlic (2 cloves crushed)

Vegetable oil (1 T)

Chicken breast (2 halved)

How's it Made

Coat a pan in the oil and place it on the stove above a burner that has been turned to a high/medium heat.

Add in the garlic, pepper, salt, pepper flakes and chicken before letting everything cook for 5 minutes.

Add in the tomatoes and cook for 5 minutes more.

Mix in the green beans before placing a lid on the pan, turning the heat to low/medium and letting it simmer for 15 minutes.

Serve hot and enjoy.

Pesto Pizza

Ingredients

Kalamata olives (8 pitted)

Tomatoes (2 chopped)

Feta cheese (.5 cups)

Pita (2)

Pesto (2 T)

How's it Made

Ensure your oven is heated to 350 degrees Fahrenheit.

Combine all ingredients before adding them to a baking sheet.

Bake pitas for 6 minutes, serve and enjoy.

Day 7

Breakfast Wrap

Ingredients

Spinach leaves (1 cup chopped)

Tomato chutney (4 T)

Feta cheese (4 T crumbled)

Tortillas (4)

Water (1 T)

Garlic chipotle seasoning (.25 tsp.)

Eggs (4 beaten)

Olive oil (1 T)

How's it Made

Coat a pan in the oil and place it on the stove above a burner that has been turned to a high/medium heat.

Add in the water, seasonings as need and eggs before scrambling the eggs and letting them cook for 3 minutes.

Add all of the ingredients to the tortillas and roll them into burritos.

Place each burrito on the skillet for 1 minute until burrito is crisp.

Serve warm and enjoy.

Lentil Soup

Ingredients

Red wine vinegar (1 tsp.)

Olive oil (1 tsp.)

Pepper and salt (to taste)

Tomato paste (1 T)

Bay leaves (2)

Rosemary (1 pinch crushed)

Oregano (1 pinch)

Water (1 quart)

Carrot (1 chopped)

Onion (1 minced)

Garlic (1 T minced)

Olive oil (.25 cups)

Lentils (8 oz.)

How's it Made

In a saucepan, add the lintels and cover them in an inch of water before letting the water boil and cooking for 10 minutes.

Coat a pan in the oil and place it on the stove above a burner that has been turned to a medium heat.

Mix in the carrot, onion and garlic and let them cook for 5 minutes.

Add in the bay leaves, rosemary, oregano and water before letting it boil.

Turn the heat to low/medium, add a lid to the pan and let it cook for 10 minutes.

Add in the pepper, salt and tomato paste before covering again and letting it simmer for 30 minutes, stirring every 10 minutes.

Add olive oil and vinegar to taste, serve and enjoy.

Eggplant Pasta

Ingredients

Basil (.5 cups)

Buffalo mozzarella cheese (.5 lbs. cubed)

Salt and pepper (to taste)

Sugar (1 tsp.)

Red wine vinegar (1 T)

Tomatoes (18 oz. crushed)

Oregano (2 tsp.)

Garlic (3 cloves minced)

Onion (1 chopped)

Olive oil (3 T divided)

Pappardelle pasta (9 oz.)

Eggplant (1 sliced)

How's it Made

In a colander, add the sliced eggplant and salt to taste. Let it sit for 10 minutes before cubing the eggplant.

Add water and salt to a large pot and place it on a burner turned to high until the water boils, add in the pasta and let it cook for 10 minutes.

Coat a pan in 1.5 T oil and place it on the stove above a burner that has been turned to a medium heat.

Add in the eggplant and let it cook for 5 minutes before removing it from the skillet.

Add the rest of the oil to the skillet before adding in the garlic and onion and letting them cook for 10 minutes.

Add the eggplant back to the skillet and let everything cook for an extra minute.

Add in the salt, pepper, sugar, vinegar and tomatoes before placing a lid on the skillet and letting everything cook for 10 minutes.

Combine ingredients, serve hot and enjoy.

Week 3

I nclude a snack of your choice during the day when you get hungry. If you don't feel hungry between meals, skip it.

Day 1

Grecian Breakfast Sandwich

Ingredients

Feta cheese (4 T)

Tomato (1 sliced)

Baby spinach (2 cups)

Eggs (4)

Rosemary (1 T)

Olive oil (4 T)

Multigrain sandwich thins (4)

How's it made

Ensure your oven is preheated to 375 degrees Fahrenheit

Brush the sandwich thins with olive oil before adding them to a baking sheet and letting them bake for 5 minutes.

Coat a pan in the oil and place it on the stove above a burner that has been turned to a high/medium heat.

Add the eggs to the pan and let them cook for 60 seconds. Let the yolks break and then flip the eggs and cook for an additional 60 seconds.

Add all ingredients to sandwich thins, serve warm and enjoy.

Tabbouleh

Ingredients

Salt and pepper (to taste)

Cucumber (1 peeled, seeded, chopped)

Tomatoes (3 chopped)

Mint (.25 cups chopped)

Parsley (1 cup chopped)

Green onions (1 cup chopped)

Lemon juice (.3 cups)

Olive oil (.3 cups)

Water (1.5 cups boiling)

Bulgur (1 cup)

How's it Made

Add the bulgur to the water, cover the pot and let it sit for 60 minutes.

Mix in the cucumber, tomatoes, mint, parsley, onions, lemon juice and oil before seasoning as needed.

Add the lid back on and let it sit in the refrigerator for at least 60 minutes before serving.

Veggie Cakes

Ingredients

Salt and pepper (to taste)

Walnuts (2 T chopped)

Eggs (3 beaten)

Sun dried tomatoes (.25 cups)

Almond flour (.3 cups)

Kalamata olives (.3 cups, sliced pitted)

Artichoke hearts (.3 cups)

Parsnip (1 grated)

Spinach (3 cups)

Garlic (3 cloves chopped)

Onion (1 cup chopped)

Olive oil (.25 cups divided)

How's it Made

Coat a pan in half the oil and place it on the stove above a burner that has been turned to a medium heat.

Add in the garlic and onion and let them cook for 5 minutes.

Add in the spinach and let it also cook for 5 minutes.

Add the results to a large and let them cool.

Into the bowl, add the remainder of the ingredients before combining well and forming the results into circles.

Add the remainder of the oil to the pan and let the circles cook for 5 minutes per side.

Serve hot and enjoy.

Day 2

Eggs Mediterranean Style

Ingredients

Feta cheese (3 oz.)

Eggs (6)

Sun dried tomatoes (.3 cups julienned)

Garlic (1 clove minced)

Olive oil (1 T)

Butter (1 T)

Onion (1.5 sliced, halved)

How's it Made

Coat a pan in the oil, add in the butter, and place it on the stove above a burner that has been turned to a medium heat.

Mix in the onions and coat them in butter and oil. Reduce heat and let them cook for 60 minutes, stirring 6 times throughout.

Mix in the sun dried tomatoes and the garlic before letting it cook for 2 minutes.

Ensure everything is well packed in the pan before adding the eggs, pepper and salt to taste and the feta cheese. Add a lid and let everything cook for 10 minutes.

Serve warm and enjoy.

Sausage Marsala

Ingredients

Pepper and salt (to taste)

Oregano (1 pinch)

Italian diced tomatoes (1 14.5 oz. can)

Marsala wine (1 T)

Red bell pepper (1 sliced)

Green bell pepper (1 sliced)

Onion (.5 sliced)

Garlic (1 clove minced)

Water (.3 cups)

Italian sausage (1 lb.)

Farfalle pasta (16 oz.)

How's it Made

Add a pinch of salt to a pot of water and let it boil before adding in the pasta and letting it cook for 8 minutes.

Add the water and the sausage to a skillet before placing it over a burner turned to a medium/high heat. Add a lid to the skillet and let it cook for 5 minutes. Slice after draining.

Add the wine, peppers, onions, garlic and sausage to the skillet before turning the burner to a high/medium heat and cooking the sausage completely.

Add in the oregano, pepper, salt and tomatoes before letting everything cook for an additional 2 minutes.

Add to pasta serve and enjoy.

Grilled Pork Chops

Ingredients

Olive oil (.3 cups)

Pork rib chops (4, .5-inch thick)

Salt (1.5 tsp.)

Bay leaf (1 crumbled)

Sugar (.5 tsp.)

Fennel seed (1 tsp. crushed)

Thyme (1 tsp.)

Rosemary leaves (2 tsp. crumbled)

Sage (2 tsp. crumbled)

How's it Made

Combine the salt, bay leaf, sugar, fennel seed, thyme, rosemary and sage together in a small bowl.

Rub the pork chops thoroughly with the results.

Heat your grill to a medium heat and add oil to it.

Grill the pork chops for 4 minutes per side and the internal temperature reads at least 145 degrees Fahrenheit.

Day 3

Breakfast Quinoa

Ingredients

Apricots (5 dried, chopped)

Dates (2 chopped, pitted)

Honey (2 T)

Vanilla extract (1 tsp.)

Sea salt (1 tsp.)

Milk (2 cups)

Quinoa (1 cup)

Cinnamon (1 tsp.)

How's it Made

Add the almonds to a pan and place the pan over a burner turned to a medium heat. Let them cook for 3 minutes and remove them from the pan.

Add the quinoa and cinnamon to the pan and letting it warm for 60 seconds.

Mix in the sea salt and milk before letting everything boil before turning the heat to low.

Add a lid to the pan and let it cook for 15 minutes.

Mix all of the ingredients together, serve warm and enjoy.

Chickpea Salad

Ingredients

Lemon juice (1 lemon)

Olive oil (2 T)

Parsley (1 T chopped)

Garlic (1 clove minced)

Onion (1 chopped)

Green bell pepper (.5 diced)

Roma tomato (1 diced)

Garbanzo beans (15 oz. can drained)

How's it Made

Combine all of the ingredients together in a large bowl, chill prior to serving.

Paprika Chicken

Ingredients

Salt and pepper (to taste)

Paprika (1 pinch)

Chili paste (to taste)

Ketchup (1 T)

Sherry vinegar (2 T)

Olive oil (.25 cups)

Chicken (8 pieces)

Cayenne pepper (1 pinch)

Olive oil (2 T +.25 cups)

Paprika (3 T)

Garlic (3 cloves)

Yogurt (6 T)

How's it Made

In a large bowl, combine the cayenne pepper, chili paste, 2 T olive oil, paprika, garlic and yogurt together and mix well.

Coat the chicken in the results before covering the bowl and leaving the chicken in the refrigerator for 3 hours.

Heat your grill to a medium heat and add oil to it as needed.

In a small bowl, add the seasonings as desired as well as ketchup, vinegar and olive oil.

Grill the chicken for 5 minutes per side with the grill closed. The chicken's internal temperature should read 180 degrees Fahrenheit.

Serve hot and enjoy.

Day 4

Breakfast Potatoes

Smoked paprika (.25 tsp.)

Cinnamon (.25 tsp.)

Oregano (.5 tsp.)

Rosemary leaves (.25 tsp crushed)

Sea salt (.5 tsp.)

Butter 91 T)

Sunflower oil (1 T)

Potato (1 diced)

How's it Made

Add the sea salt, rosemary leaves, oregano, cinnamon and paprika to a spice grinder and grind as desired.

Coat a pan in the butter and place it on the stove above a burner that has been turned to a high/medium heat.

Add in the potatoes and let them cook for 5 minutes.

Drain potatoes, cover in salt mixture, serve hot and enjoy.

Veggie Pasta

Ingredients

Tapenade (2 T)

Parmesan cheese (.25 cups grated)

Fettuccini noodles (8 oz.)

Olive oil (2 T)

Oregano (.5 tsp. chopped)

Rosemary (.5 tsp. chopped)

Tomato (1 quartered)

Garlic (10 cloves chopped, roasted)

Cremini mushrooms (.25 lbs. sliced)

Red bell pepper (2 sliced)

Asparagus (.25 lbs. sliced)

How's it Made

Ensure your oven is preheated to 350 degrees Fahrenheit.

Add tomato, garlic, mushrooms, bell pepper and asparagus together in a roasting pan before adding the olive oil, oregano and rosemary.

Add the roasting pan to the oven and let it bake for 15 minutes.

Add salt and water to a pot before bringing it to a boil. Once it boils, add in the pasta and let it cook for 8 minutes.

Add vegetables, tapenade and parmesan cheese to the pasta and mix well.

Serve warm and enjoy.

Stuffed Zucchini

Ingredients

Mozzarella (.75 cups shredded)

Bread crumbs (.75 cups)

Mint leaves (.5 cups)

Water (.25 cups)

Pine nuts (.5 cups)

Feta cheese (.75 cups)

Tomatoes (2 chopped)

Tomato sauce (16 oz.)

Pepper and salt (to taste)

Ground lamb (1 lb.)

Chopped garlic (1 T)

Sweet onion (1 chopped)

Olive oil (1 T)

Zucchini (1 sliced vertically)

How's it Made

Ensure your oven is preheated to 450 degrees Fahrenheit.

Remove half of the zucchini meat from the inside of the zucchini.

Cube the results, removing the seeds.

Coat a pan in the oil and place it on the stove above a burner that has been turned to a medium heat.

Add in the garlic and the onion and let them cook for 5 minutes.

Mix in the lamb and let it cook for 5 minutes before adding in the zucchini cubes, turning the heat to low/medium and letting it simmer for 3 minutes.

Add mint leaves, pine nuts, feta cheese, tomatoes and tomato sauce to the zucchini bowls, add the bowls to a baking dish along with the water.

Add the baking dish to the oven and let it cook for 30 minutes before adding in the remaining ingredients and cooking for an additional 10 minutes.

Serve hot and enjoy.

Day 5

Breakfast Casserole

Ingredients

Garlic (2 cloves minced)

Mushrooms (.6 cups sliced)

Tomatoes (2 diced)

Artichoke hearts (4, chopped)

Scallions (.5 cups)

Spinach (4 oz.)

Feta cheese (.5 cups)

Garlic powder (.25 tsp.)

Pepper (.25 tsp.)

Sea salt (1 tsp.)

Oregano (1 T chopped)

Parmesan cheese (2 T)

Almond milk (.25 cups)

Eggs whites (4)

Eggs (8)

How's it Made

Ensure your oven is preheated to 375 degrees Fahrenheit.

Combine the garlic powder, pepper, salt, oregano, parmesan, milk, egg white and eggs together in a mixing bowl.

Coat a baking pan with cooking spray and layer in the garlic, mushrooms, tomatoes, artichokes, scallions and spinach before topping with the egg. Rotate the dish to ensure the egg penetrates completely.

Add to oven and let bake for 30 minutes.

Let cool for 10 minutes prior to serving.

Figs Stuffed with Goat Cheese

Ingredients

Honey (.5 cups)

Grape leaves (8 rinsed, drained)

Goat cheese (.5 cups softened)

Figs (8 fresh)

How's it Made

Ensure your grill is heated to a medium heat.

Slice a space in each fig large enough to fit a pastry bag nozzle.

Add the goat cheese to the pastry bag and then fill each fig with goat cheese.

Wrap the figs in the grape leaves before adding the figs to skewers, two figs per skewer.

Add the figs to the grill and let them cook for 2 minutes, turning at one minute.

Top with honey, serve warm and enjoy.

Lemon Chicken

Ingredients

Lemon (1 sliced)

Red onion (1 wedged)

Red bell pepper (1 chopped)

Baby red potatoes (8 halved)

Chicken breast (2 halved)

Pepper and salt (to taste)

Oregano (1 T)

Garlic (4 cloves pressed)

Lemon zest (2 T)

Lemon juice (2 T)

Olive oil (.25 cups)

How's it Made

Ensure your oven is heated to 400 degrees Fahrenheit.

In a small bowl, mix the salt, pepper, oregano, garlic, lemon zest, lemon juice and olive oil.

Add the chicken to a baking dish before coating it in the lemon mixture.

In a large bowl, add the lemon slices, red onions, red bell peppers and potatoes before covering in the remaining lemon mixture.

Add the everything to the baking dish before placing it in the oven and letting it cook for 30 minutes.

Serve hot and enjoy.

Day 6

Pasta Frittata

Ingredients

Basil (.25 cups chopped)

Penne pasta (3 cups)

Feta cheese (.25 cups)

Sun dried tomatoes (.25 cups chopped)

Red pepper flakes (.25 tsp.)

Salt (.25 tsp.)

Milk (.5 cups)

Eggs (6)

Spinach (2 cups chopped)

Red onion (1 chopped)

Garlic (2 cloves minced)

Olive Oil (2 T divided)

How's it Made

Ensure your oven is preheated to 400 degrees Fahrenheit.

Coat a pan in half the oil and place it on the stove above a burner that has been turned to a high/medium heat.

Add in the onion and let it sauté for 5 minutes.

Add in the garlic and let it cook for half a minute before mixing in the spinach and letting it wilt.

Remove the skillet from the burner and let it sit for 5 minutes.

Combine the red pepper, salt, milk and eggs together before mixing in the cooled skillet vegetables, basil, pasta, feta and tomatoes.

Add the rest of the oil to the pan and set it on a burner turned to a medium heat. Add the egg mix to the pan and let it cook for 2 minutes.

Add the pan to the oven and let it cook for 10 minutes.

Let cool for 5 minutes prior to serving.

Mediterranean Salad Medley

Ingredients

Salt and pepper (to taste)

Balsamic vinegar (1 T)

Olive oil (2 T)

Basil leaves (.5 cups torn)

Kalamata olives (.25 cups sliced)

Feta cheese (2 oz. crumbled)

Vegetable combination (4 cups your choice chopped)

How's it Made

Mix all of the ingredients together in a large bowl, serve and enjoy.

Vegetable stew

Ingredients

Parsley (1 cup chopped)

Rosemary (1 T chopped)

Chickpeas (15 oz. can)

Kalamata olives (.5 cups sliced, pitted)

Tomatoes (28 oz. crushed)

Eggplant (1 cubed)

Mushrooms (1 cup)

Garlic cloves (2 crushed)

Green pepper (2 cups chopped)

Red onion (1 cup chopped)

Olive oil (2 T divided)

How's it Made

Coat a pan in half of the oil and place it on the stove above a burner that has been turned to a high/medium heat.

Add in the pepper and onion and let them cook for 10 minutes.

Add in the remainder of the oil as well as the eggplant, mushrooms and garlic. Let the pan simmer for 15 minutes.

Mix in the chickpeas, rosemary and olives before letting everything simmer for another 10 minutes.

Add in the parsley, serve warm and enjoy.

Day 7

Breakfast Enchilada

Ingredients

Black olives (6 sliced)

Tomatoes (.5 cups sliced)

Salt (.75 tsp.)

Green chilies (4.5 oz. can)

Cheddar cheese (2 cups shredded)

Milk (3 cups)

Flour (.3 cups)

Butter (.3 cups)

Mexican cheese (1 cup shredded)

Tortillas (8)

Pepper (.5 tsp.)

Salt (.75 tsp.)

Eggs (14)

Cilantro (2 T)

Scallions (4 sliced)

Butter (2 T)

Breakfast soy (8 oz. cooked)

How's it Made

Add butter to a pan placed over a burner turned to a medium heat and add in flour, stirring until smooth. Let the flour cook for 60 seconds.

Add in the milk and stirring constantly for 5 minutes.

Remove the pan from the burner before mixing in the salt, chili and cheese to finish sauce.

Add fresh butter to the pan before adding in the cilantro and scallions and letting them sauté. Add in the pepper, salt and eggs and let the eggs start to cook.

Let the eggs cook most of the way before adding in the cheese and the breakfast soy.

Finish cooking the eggs, add everything to the tortillas and cover with sauce.

Serve hot and enjoy.

Grecian Chicken Soup

Ingredients

Chicken stock (1.5 cups)

Bay leaves (2)

Oregano (1 pinch)

Parsley (2 T chopped)

Tomato sauce (1 cup)

Red wine (.5 cups)

Garlic (2 cloves chopped)

Whole chicken (4 lbs. separated)

Butter (2 tsp.)

Olive oil (1 cup)

Shallots (10 peeled)

How's it made

Add a pinch of salt and water to a large pot and let it boil.

Mix in the shallots and let them cook for 3 minutes then drain them and place them in cold water to prevent them from cooking further.

Add the butter and olive oil to a large skillet and let it heat until the butter melts.

Add in the chicken and the shallots, turning the chicken as needed for 15 minutes.

Mix in the garlic and let everything cook for 3 additional minutes.

Add the bay leaves, oregano, pepper, salt, parsley, tomato sauce and the red wine before mixing well.

Cover the skillet and let it simmer on a low/medium heat for 50 minutes

Serve hot and enjoy.

Eggplant Chicken

Ingredients

Pepper and salt to taste

Oregano (2 tsp.)

Water (.5 cups)

Tomato paste (2 T)

Onion (1 diced)

Chicken breast (6 halves)

Olive oil (3 T0

Eggplants (3 peel, sliced)

How's it Made

Fill a pot with water, add a pinch of salt and add in the eggplant and let it sit for 30 minutes.

Coat the eggplant in olive oil before adding it to a pan and placing the pan over a burner turned to a medium heat. Sauté it and add it to a baking dish.

Add in the onion and well as the chicken before mixing in the water and tomato paste before adding a lid to the pan and turning the heat to low before letting everything cook for 10 minutes.

Ensure your oven is heated to 400 degrees Fahrenheit.

Add the remainder of the ingredients to the baking pan before seasoning as desired and wrapping everything in aluminum foil.

Bake for 20 minutes, serve hot and enjoy.

Week 4

I nclude a snack of your choice during the day when you get hungry. If you don't feel hungry between meals, skip it.

Day 1

Mediterranean Omelet

Ingredients

Olive oil (1 T)

Mediterranean spice seasoning (2 T)

Feta cheese crumble (.25 cups)

Spinach (.3 cups)

Bella mushrooms (.3 cups sliced)

Grape tomatoes (.3 cups chopped)

Eggs (2)

How's it Made

Add the eggs to a mixing bowl and whisk well.

Add the oil to a pan and place it on a burner turned to a medium heat.

Add the eggs and let each side cook for 2 minutes.

Add in the remaining ingredients and fold over when desired.

Serve warm and enjoy.

Mediterranean Wrap

Ingredients

Avocado (1 sliced)

Basil pesto (.25 cups)

Goat cheese (.25 cups)

Tortillas (4)

Salt and pepper (to taste)

Olive oil (1 T)

Red bell pepper (1 sliced)

Mushrooms (.25 lbs. sliced)

Eggplant (1 sliced)

Zucchini (1 sliced)

Red onion (1 sliced)

How's it Made

Add the bell pepper, mushrooms, eggplant, zucchini and onion to a plastic container with a well-fitting lid. Add in the pepper, salt and olive oil, close the container and coat well by shaking.

Add a skillet to a burner turned to a medium heat. Add in the vegetables and let them cook for 10 minutes stirring every 3 minutes.

Add the results to the tortillas, serve and enjoy.

Puff Pastry Chicken

Ingredients

Puff pastry sheet (1 halved)

Feta cheese (.25 cups crumbled)

Sun dried tomatoes (.3 cups)

Basil pesto (2 T)

Chicken breast (2 halved)

Spinach (2 cups)

Egg yolk (1)

Garlic (3 T)

How's it Made

Combine the egg yolk and garlic in a bowl before adding the chicken to a baking dish and adding the egg and garlic on top of it. Cover the dish and leave it in the refrigerator overnight.

Ensure your oven is heat to 374 degrees Fahrenheit.

Add the ingredients to the pastry before placing them on a baking sheet and placing the sheet in the oven for 35 minutes.

Day 2

Spanakopita

Ingredients

Olive oil (2 tsp.)

Dill 92 T)

Scallions (2 sliced)

Feta cheese (.5 cups)

Eggs (4)

Spinach (.25 cups cooked)

How's it Made

Ensure your boiler is preheated and the rack is 4 inches away.

Combine the spinach, dill, scallions, feta and eggs together in a mixing bowl.

Coat a pan in the oil and place it on the stove above a burner that has been turned to a medium heat.

Add the results of the bowl to the pan and let it cook for 3 minutes.

Place the pan underneath the boiler and let it cook for 2 minutes.

Serve warm and enjoy.

Fish Soup

Ingredients

Cod (1 lb. cubed)

Shrimp (1 lb. deveined, peeled)

Salt and pepper (to taste)

Fennel seed (.25 tsp. crushed)

Basil (1 tsp.)

Bay leaves (2)

Dry white wine (.5 cups)

Orange Juice (.5 cups)

Black olives (.25 cups sliced)

Mushrooms (2.5 oz.)

Tomato sauce (8 oz.)

Chicken broth (28 oz.)

Tomatoes (14.5 oz. can diced, drained)

Garlic (2 cloves minced)

Bell pepper (.5 chopped)

Onion (1 chopped)

How's it Made

Add the pepper, fennel, basil, bay, wine, juice, olives, mushroom, tomato sauce, chicken broth, tomatoes, garlic, bell pepper and onion into a crockpot, cover it and let everything cook on a low temperature for 4 hours.

Add in the cod as well as the shrimp, return the lid to the crockpot and let it cook until the shrimp turn opaque which should take 20 minutes.

Serve hot and enjoy.

Fish Cakes

Ingredients

Flour (4 T)

Shrimp (6.5 oz.)

Tuna (9 oz.)

Bread crumbs (.5 cups)

Italian seasoning (1 T)

Chili peppers (2 seeded)

Basil (6 leaves)

Egg (1)

Sun dried tomatoes (5 chopped)

Garlic (4 cloves)

Onion (.5)

Scallops (6 oz.)

Olive oil (4 T)

How's it Made

Coat a pan in 1 T oil and place it on the stove above a burner that has been turned to a high/medium heat.

Add in the scallops and let them cook until they are completely white.

In a food processor, mix in 1 T olive oil, the egg, tomatoes, garlic and onion before adding in the seasoning, chilies, basil and parsley and process on the medium setting.

Add in the shrimp, scallops and tuna and process on a low setting.

Add in the breadcrumbs and keep processing until everything binds together.

Make the results into patties before adding them to a plate and placing the plate in the refrigerator for at least 2 hours.

Coat a pan in the remaining oil and place it on the stove above a burner that has been turned to a medium heat.

Cook the patties in the pan until both sides have turned a golden brown.

Day 3

Chickpea Cucumber Breakfast

Ingredients

Dill (2 T)

Feta cheese (2 T)

Cucumber (.5 cups)

Kalamata olives (2 pitted, chopped)

Red bell peppers (2 T chopped)

Chickpeas (.5 cups)

Salt and pepper (to taste)

Red wine vinegar (1.5 tsp.)

Olive oil (1.5 tsp.)

How's it Made

In a medium bowl, combine the olive oil, vinegar and salt and pepper before mixing well. Add in the olives, peppers and chickpeas before coating well.

Add in the cucumber slices, mix well, serve and enjoy.

Bean Salad

Ingredients

Salt (.5 tsp.)

Olive oil (3 T)

Capers (1 tsp.)

Parsley (.5 cups chopped)

Red onion (.25 cups)

Tomato (1 chopped)

Lemon zest (1 lemon)

Lemon juice (1 lemon)

Kidney beans (15 oz. drained)

Garbanzo beans (15.5 oz. drained)

How's it made

Combine all of the ingredients together in a large bowl before covering the bowl and letting it sit in the refrigerator for at least 3 hours, stirring twice per hour prior to serving.

Seafood Medley

Ingredients

Parsley (6 sprigs)

Olive oil (2 T)

Pepper and salt (to taste)

Sea bass filets (6, 6 oz.)

Mussels (20)

Littleneck clams (20)

Oysters (10)

Thyme (.5 bunches chopped)

Fennel bulbs (6 halved)

Sundried tomatoes (.5 cups chopped)

Garlic (6 cloves minced)

Olive oil (2 T)

Saffron (1 T)

Peppercorn (1 tsp.)

Bay leaves (2)

Tarragon (.5 bunches)

Chicken stock (3 cups)

White wine (1 cup)

Tomato paste (.5 cups)

Tomatoes (2 chopped)

Carrots (2 chopped)

Onions (2 chopped)

Milk (3 cups)

Baby squid (20)

How's it Made

Add the milk and the squid to a pot and let it soak for 4 hours.

Coat a pan in 2 T oil and place it on the stove above a burner that has been turned to a high/medium heat.

Add in the fennel, tomatoes, carrots, onions and garlic before letting them cook for 10 minutes.

Add in the tomato paste and let it cook for 10 minutes.

Increase the heat before adding in the wine and letting the pan boil.

Add in the saffron, peppercorns, bay leaves, thyme, tarragon, parsley and chicken stock and let everything boil before turning the burner to a medium heat and letting it simmer for 15 minutes.

Separate the solids and liquids.

Coat a pan in 2 T oil and place it on the stove above a burner that has been turned to a high/medium heat.

Add in the garlic and let it cook for 45 seconds before mixing in the tomatoes and the fell and letting them cook for 3 minutes.

Add the broth to the pan and let it boil before adding in the oysters and letting it cook for 60 seconds.

Add the mussels and clams, add a lid to the pan and let it cook for 5 minutes.

Add pepper and salt to the bass before coating a pan in the remaining oil and place it on the stove above a burner that has been turned to a high/medium heat.

Cook the fish, combine all of the ingredients, serve hot and enjoy.

Day 4

Breakfast Pizza

Ingredients

Oregano (.25 tsp.)

Spike seasoning (.5 tsp.)

Mozzarella (1 oz.)

Black olives (6 sliced)

Pepperoni (6 slices)

Eggs (2 beaten)

Olive oil (1 tsp.)

How's it Made

Ensure your broiler is preheated.

Coat a pan in the oil and place it on the stove above a burner that has been turned to a medium heat.

Add the eggs to the pan and season them to taste, let them cook for 2 minutes.

Add the remaining ingredients to the top of the eggs and put a lid on the pan before letting it cook for 3 minutes.

Remove the pan from the burner and place it underneath the broiler for 2 minutes.

Serve hot and enjoy.

Pasta Salad

Ingredients

Pepper and salt (to taste)

Parmesan cheese (.5 cups grated)

Garbanzo beans (15 oz. rinsed, drained)

Scallions (1 bunch chopped)

Parsley (2 T)

Oregano (2 T)

Oil cured olives (.5 cups)

Olive oil (2 T)

Rotelle pasta (16 oz.)

How's it Made

Add salt and water to a large pot before waiting for the water to boil and adding the pasta and letting it cook for 10 minutes.

Coat a pan in the oil and place it on the stove above a burner that has been turned to a low/medium heat.

Add in the chickpeas, scallions, parsley, oregano and olives and let them cook for 20 minutes.

Combine the chickpeas with the pasta before mixing in the seasoning, cheese and vinegar.

Let the results cool overnight prior to serving.

Lentil/Lamb Stew

Ingredients

Lemon zest (1 lemon)

Lemon juice (1 lemon)

Spinach (2 cups chopped)

Basil (.5 tsp.)

Sage (.5 tsp.)

Thyme (.5 tsp.)

Carrots (sliced, peeled)

Chicken broth (2 cups)

Lentils (1 cup)

Garlic (4 cloves minced)

Onion (1 chopped)

Salt and pepper (to taste)

Lamb shoulder (1. 5 lbs. cubed)

Olive oil (1 T)

Ricotta cheese salata (.5 cups)

How's it Made

Add the oil to a large pot before placing it over a burner turned to a high/medium heat.

Add in the bones and lamb bits before letting them cook for 3 minutes.

Add in the seasoning as well as the garlic and onion and cook for 2 minutes.

Add in the broth, basil, sage, thyme, carrots and tomatoes before letting the lentil cook for 20 minutes.

Remove the bones before adding the spinach and letting everything cook for 5 minutes.

Add in the lemon juice and zest, top with cheese, serve hot and enjoy.

Day 5

Sausage Queso

Ingredients

Green onions (4 sliced)

Cream of Chicken Soup (1 can)

Black olives (1 cup chopped)

Tomatoes and Green Chilies (2 cans)

Onion (1 chopped)

Velveeta cheese (2 lbs.)

Breakfast sausage (2 lbs. browned)

How's it made

Add all ingredients to a crockpot and stir well.

Heat on a low heat until cheese has melted.

Serve and enjoy.

Romaine with Anchovy Dressing

Ingredients

Pepper and salt (to taste)

Parmesan cheese (.25 lbs. grated)

Romaine lettuce (1 head cut into .5 inch pieces)

Olive oil (.25 cups)

Lemon juice (2 tsp.)

Anchovy fillet (2)

Garlic (1 clove minced)

How's it made

Add the lemon juice, anchovies and garlic to a blender and blend well, as the blender is blending, mix in the oil and pepper and salt as needed.

Add all of the ingredients together, mix well to coat, serve and enjoy.

Mediterranean Trout

Ingredients

White wine (2 T dry)

Parsley (1 bunch chopped)

Capers 91 T)

Tomatoes (4 chopped)

Kalamata olives (2 T)

Anchovy fillets (3 chopped)

Onions (2 sliced)

Bell pepper (1 yellow)

Salt and pepper (to taste)

Italian seasoning (2 T)

Trout fillet (4)

Olive oil (2 T)

Potatoes (6 diced)

How's it Made

Add the potatoes to a pot, fill with water and a pinch of salt. Let the water boil and cook the potatoes for 8 minutes. Drain the potatoes

Coat a pan in the oil and place it on the stove above a burner that has been turned to a high/medium heat.

Add the fish and seasonings to the pan before letting it cook for 10 minutes.

Flip the fillets before adding the onions and peppers and letting them cook for 5 minutes.

Add in the parsley, capers, tomatoes, olive and anchovies before adding in the whine and letting everything cook for 5 minutes.

Combine all of the ingredients, serve hot and enjoy.

Day 6

Mediterranean Quiche

Ingredients

Goat cheese (4 oz. crumbled)

Red pepper (.5 tsp.)

Gruyere (1.5 cups grated)

Half-and-half (1.25 cups)

Eggs (3)

Black pepper (.25 tsp.)

Salt (.5 tsp.)

Thyme (2 tsp.)

Basil (2 oz.)

Sun dried tomatoes (4 oz.)

Garlic (1 clove minced)

Red pepper (1 diced)

Zucchini (1 diced)

Onion (1 diced)

Butter (2 T)

Pie crusts (2)

How's it Made

Ensure your oven is preheated to 375 degrees Fahrenheit.

Coat a pan in the butter and place it on the stove above a burner that has been turned to a high/medium heat.

Mix in the onions and let them cook for 5 minutes.

Mix in the zucchini and let it cook for 5 minutes.

Add in the red pepper and let everything cook for 4 more minutes.

Mix in the garlic and let it cook for 60 seconds.

Remove the pan from the burner and add in the pepper, salt, thyme, basil and tomatoes.

Combine the red pepper, gruyere, pepper, salt, half and half and eggs together in a large bowl.

Add the results of the bowl to the pan and add the cheese on top.

Place the pan in the oven and let it bake for 45 minutes.

Cool for 30 minutes, serve, enjoy.

Grecian Farfalle

Ingredients

Red wine (.5 cups)

Olive oil (.5 cups)

Tomato (1 cup diced)

Parmesan cheese (.5 cups)

Garlic (2 cloves minced)

Pine nuts (.5 cups)

Basil (.25 cups chopped)

Chorizo sausage (1 lb. crumbled)

Farfalle pasta (12 oz.)

How's it Made

Add salt and water to a pot before letting it boil and adding the pasta and letting it cook for 10 minutes.

Coat a pan in oil and place it on the stove above a burner that has been turned to a high/medium heat.

Brown the sausage before adding in the nuts and letting them brown. Mix in the garlic before removing the pan from the heat.

Combine the vinegar and olive oil in a small bowl and mix well.

Combine all of the ingredients, serve hot and enjoy.

Stuffed Swordfish

Ingredients

Feta (.25 cups crumbled)

Garlic (1 clove minced)

Olive oil (1 tsp.)

Spinach (2 cups)

Lemon juice (1 T)

Olive Oil (1 T)

Swordfish Steak (8 oz.)

How's it Made

Heat your grill to a high heat before oiling it as needed.

Add a small pocket to the steak.

Combine the lemon juice and olive oil before applying that to the fish.

Coat a pan in the oil and place it on the stove above a burner that has been turned to a medium heat before adding the spinach and letting it cook for 5 minutes.

Add the spinach and the cheese to the fish pocket before letting it grill for 8 minutes on each side.

Serve hot and enjoy.

Day 7

Maacouda

Ingredients

Salt (.5 tsp.)

Eggs (6 beaten)

Mint (6 leaves crushed)

Black olives (.25 cups)

Olive oil (1 T)

Onion (1 sliced)

Potatoes (1 lb. mashed)

How's it made

Coat a pan in the oil and place it on the stove above a burner that has been turned to a medium heat.

Add in the onions and cook for 20 minutes.

Ensure the oven is preheated to 450 degrees Fahrenheit.

Grease a baking pan

Add the eggs to the potatoes before mixing well.

Mix in the mint, olive and onions.

Add the results to the dish and let it bake in the oven for 20 minutes.

Serve hot and enjoy.

Brown Rice Salad

Feta Cheese (.25 cups)

Pepper and salt (to taste)

Dijon mustard (1.25 tsp.)

Balsamic vinegar (.25 cups)

Sweet onion (.25)

Raisins (.5 cups)

Peas (1 cup)

Red bell pepper (1 sliced)

Water (3 cups)

Vegetable oil (.5 cups)

How's it Made

Add the water and rice to a saucepan and place it on a burner turned to a high heat.

Let it boil before reducing the heat to low/medium, placing the lid on the saucepan and let it simmer for 45 minutes.

In a large bowl, add the olives, onion, raisins, peas and bell peppers.

In a separate bowl, combine the mustard, vinegar, and vegetable oil and mix well.

Combine all ingredients, serve and enjoy.

Pepperoncini Chicken

Ingredients

Paprika (.5 tsp.)

Sour cream (1 cup)

Lemon juice (.5 cups)

Lemon zest (.5 tsp.)

Salt and pepper (to taste)

Paprika (1.5 tsp.)

Chicken legs (3.5 lbs.)

Garlic (8 cloves minced)

Kalamata olives (1 cup sliced)

Pepperoncini peppers (12)

How's it Made

In a slow cooker combine all of the ingredients except for the sour cream and let it cook on low for 6 hours.

Remove fat for slow cooker before adding in sour cream and mixing well. Cook for 8 minutes and season as desired.

Serve hot and enjoy.

Snacks

Olives with Feta

Ingredients

Pepper/red pepper (to taste)

Rosemary (1 tsp. chopped)

Garlic (2 cloves sliced)

Lemon juice (1 lemon)

Lemon zest (1 lemon)

Olive oil (2 T)

Feta cheese (.5 cups)

Kalamata olives (1 cup)

How's it Made

Combine all of the ingredients and let them sit in the refrigerator for 24 hours to marinate.

Snack Pizza

Ingredients

Feta cheese (.5 cups)

Red bell peppers (.3 cups chopped)

Kalamata olives (.3 cups pitted, sliced)

Artichoke hearts (6 oz. chopped)

Mozzarella cheese (1 cup shredded)

Premade pizza dough

How's it made

Ensure your oven is heated to 400 degrees Fahrenheit.

Coat cookie sheet with cooking spray.

Add dough to sheet and shape as desired.

Bake dough for 10 minutes before adding all of the ingredients and baking for 6 additional minutes.

Mediterranean snack

Ingredients

Olives (6 pitted)

Cheese (.25 oz. slice)

Cherry tomatoes (10)

How's it Made

Eat the three ingredients at the same time

Greek Dip

Ingredients

Pita chips

Green onions (2 T chopped)

Kalamata olives (.5 cups pitted chopped)

Cucumber (.5 cups chopped)

Roma tomatoes (3 chopped)

Hummus (1 cup)

Salt (to taste)

Lemon juice (1 tsp.)

Parsley (1 T)

Feta cheese (.25 cups)

Lemon yogurt (6 oz.)

How's it made

Combine all of the ingredients and mix well, add to pita chips and enjoy.

Hard-Boiled Egg with Paprika

Ingredients

Paprika (.5 tsp.)

Kosher salt (.5 tsp.)

Olive oi (1 tsp.)

2 eggs (hard-boiled)

How to prepare

Slice the eggs in half and dip the halves in the other ingredients.

Grecian Snack Cups

Ingredients

Kalamata olives (.25 cups pitted, sliced)

Guacamole (.5 cups)

Feta cheese (.3 cups crumbled)

Sun dried tomatoes (.5 cups chopped)

Premade dinner roll dough (1 can)

How's it Made

Ensure your oven is heated to 375 degrees Fahrenheit.

Coat a muffin tin in cooking spray before adding the dinner roll dough to the muffin tins.

Add the feta and tomatoes on top of the dough before baking for 14 minutes.

Top with olives and guacamole, serve hot and enjoy.

Finger Sandwiches

Ingredients

Pepper and salt (to taste)

Basil (4 tsp. sliced)

Tomatoes (2 sliced)

Mayonnaise (8 tsp. divided)

Rye Bread (4 slices)

How's it Made

Slice out bread rounds that are equal to the width of your tomato slices.

Combine ingredients into mini sandwiches.

Hummus Nachos

Ingredients

Oregano leaves (1 T chopped)

Feta cheese (.25 cups crumbled)

Kalamata olives (.25 cups chopped, pitted)

Roma tomato (1 chopped)

Cucumber (.5 cups chopped)

Roasted red pepper hummus (8 oz.)

Pita chips

How's it Made

Ensure your oven is heated to 400 degrees Fahrenheit.

Place the chips as the bottom layer in a baking tray before topping with cheese, olives, tomato, and cucumber and baking for 5 minutes.

Top with lemon peel and oregano, serve hot and enjoy.

Olives and Herbs

Ingredients

Salt and pepper (to taste)

Garlic (1 clove crushed)

Basil (.25 tsp.)

Oregano (.25 tsp.)

Olive oil (2 tsp.)

Kalamata olives (3 cups pitted)

How's it made

Combine all ingredients, mix well, serve and enjoy.

Arancini

Ingredients

Olive oil (2 T)

Water (1 T)

Egg (1)

Bread crumbs (1.5 cups)

Flour (.5 cups)

Mozzarella cheese (4 oz. cubed)

Parmesan cheese (.5 cups grated)

Butter (1 T)

Spinach leaves (1 cup chopped)

Salt/pepper (to taste)

Chicken broth (2 cups)

White wine (.5 cups)

Rice (.75 cups)

Garlic (2 cloves chopped)

Onion (1 chopped)

How's it Made

Cover a cookie sheet in parchment paper.

Coat a pan in the oil and place it on the stove above a burner that has been turned to a high/medium heat.

Add in the onion and let it cook for 60 seconds, mix in the garlic and let it cook for 5 minutes.

Turn heat to medium before adding in the wine and rice and cooking for 5 minutes and adding in 1 cup broth and cooking for 10 minutes and repeating with the other cup of broth.

Add in the pepper, cheese, butter and spinach before adding the results to the cookie sheet.

Cover and place in the refrigerator for 90 minutes.

Cut the results in 24 squares and add cheese to each.

Roll each square into a ball before using the egg, flour and bread crumbs to coat each ball and place them on a platter.

Heat vegetable oil in a Dutch oven until it reaches 350 degrees Fahrenheit.

Fry the balls for 3 minutes, serve hot and enjoy.

Wrapped Dates

Ingredients

Pepper (to taste)

16 (dates pitted)

Prosciutto (16 slices)

How's it made

Wrap each date with prosciutto and season as needed.

Banana Gelato

Ingredients

Whipping cream (.25 cups)

Salt (.25 tsp.)

Vanilla extract (2 tsp.)

Sugar (.75 cups)

Egg Yolks (5)

Brown sugar (.25 cups)

Bananas (3 quartered, peeled)

Skim milk (1.75 cups)

How's it Made

In a large saucepan, combine the brown sugar, bananas and milk and place the pan on a burner turned to a medium heat. Add a lid to the pan, turn the heat down and let it cook for 10 minutes

Let everything cool before adding it to a blender and blending well.

Add the results back to the pan.

In a large bowl, combine the yolks and sugar.

Add half of the pan to the bowl and mix well.

Add everything back into the pan and let it cook for 2 minutes on a low heat, stirring well. Mix in the cream, salt and vanilla.

Add everything to a container and refrigerate for 48 hours before freezing.

Lemon Crème and Blueberries

Ingredients

Blueberries (2 cups)

Lemon zest (2 tsp.)

Honey (1 tsp.)

Vanilla yogurt (.75 cups)

Cream cheese (4 oz.)

How's it made

In a medium sized bowl, mix all of the ingredients together well, serve and enjoy.

Skewered Basil and Tomatoes

Ingredients

Salt and pepper (to taste)

Olive oil (to taste)

Cherry tomatoes (16)

Basil leaves (16)

Mozzarella (16 balls)

How's it Made

Add the ingredients to a skewer before drizzling olive oil on top and seasoning as desired.

Sweet Potato Fries

Ingredients

Seasoning (to taste)

Olive oil (2 T)

Sweet potatoes (2 sliced as desired)

How's it Made

Ensure your oven is heated to 425 degrees Fahrenheit.

Coat the potatoes in oil and salt before adding them to a baking sheet that has been coated in cooking spray.

Let the fries cook for 15 minutes, serve and enjoy.

Toasted Almonds, Ricotta and Cherries

Ingredients

Almonds (1 T toasted, slivered)

Ricotta (2 T)

Cherries (.75 cups pitted)

How's it Made

Add cherries to a microwaveable bowl before adding them to the microwave and heating them for 1 minutes.

Combine all of the ingredients, serve warm and enjoy.

Conclusion

Thank you again for downloading this book!

I hope this book was able to help you to gain a better understanding of the Mediterranean diet and other tips for incorporating it into your life on a regular basis.

The next step is entirely up to you. So go out there and take control of your life and reclaim your health with the Mediterranean diet!

Finally, if you enjoyed this book, then I'd like to ask you for a favor, would you be kind enough to leave a review for this book on Amazon? It'd be greatly appreciated!

Thank you and good luck!

Check Out My Other Books

Below you'll find some of my other popular books that are popular on Amazon and Kindle as well. Simply click on the links below to check them out. Alternatively, you can visit my author page on Amazon to see other work done by me.

If the links do not work, for whatever reason, you can simply search for these titles on the Amazon website to find them.

BOOKS BY LR SMITH:

Low Carb High Fat - Click here

Ketogenic Diet - Click here

Anti-Inflammatory Diet - Click here

Whole Food - Click here

Dash Diet - Click here

Bone Broth - Click here

Mediterranean Diet - Click here

www.ingramcontent.com/pod-product-compliance
Lightning Source LLC
Chambersburg PA
CBHW071359280526
45787CB00001B/382